Parenting with

Purpose

A Modern Guide to Raising Successful Children

Parenting with Purpose

A Modern Guide to Raising Successful Children

Prologue:

The day he was born, everything changed. The world shifted beneath my feet. It wasn't a gradual change; it was immediate, a tidal wave of emotions I didn't know existed. I had reached a summit I didn't even know I was climbing. In that moment, I realized that all of my choices, sacrifices, and paths had led to this: the ultimate gift of fatherhood.

Parenting, though, is never about one single moment. It's about a million little ones strung together, each choice building on the last. And there's no manual for it. You don't get handed a guidebook when you leave the hospital, telling you how to raise a successful child. Instead, you're thrown into the deep end, navigating sleepless nights, diaper changes, and your own lingering doubts. The doubts that creep in late at night—Am I doing this right? Am I enough for them?

When my wife and I venture out in public with our kids, the highest compliment we receive is when people tell us how well-behaved they are. It's those small, unexpected moments that stick with you. One that comes to mind was during a family lunch. We were out with our extended family when a grandmother approached our table. She said, "I don't know whose kids these are, but they are just wonderful. Way to go, mom and dad." I thanked her, and in that brief exchange, I felt an enormous sense of pride.

But also, underneath that pride, I felt a wave of relief wash over me. As parents, we often live in this constant state of self-questioning—Am I screwing this all up? Hearing those words from a stranger, someone who took the time to notice and acknowledge, was like a quiet confirmation that we were doing something right.

It wasn't long after that our friends started saying things that took me by surprise. The first time one of them mentioned they wanted to parent like us, I felt honored. The fifth time, it started to feel like there was something more here—something worth sharing. Friends would come over for advice, to ask about our routines, how we handled discipline, how we managed to raise kids who, at least outwardly, seemed to have it all together.

The final push came from my son. He overheard me giving some advice to a friend and, in that way only kids can, without pretense or filter, said, "You should write a book." I laughed it off at first—Sure, buddy, sounds easy enough. But he looked at me, completely serious, and said, "No, really. Think about it."

And I did.

That was the moment when it clicked. I realized that maybe, just maybe, our experiences could help other parents. Maybe sharing what worked for us—the good, the bad, the trial and error—might be worth putting into words. Not because we've figured it all out (because we haven't), but because we're still learning. And what we've learned so far has given us children who feel loved, understood, and empowered.

So, here it is. A book born from years of parenting highs and lows, from compliments received at random, from friends who trusted us enough to ask for guidance, and from a son who reminded me that sometimes, the best ideas are the ones staring you in the face.

This isn't a perfect guide to parenting—it's just our guide. But if there's one thing I've learned on this journey, it's that parenting with purpose, with intention, is the greatest gift you can give your children. And I'm here to share how we've tried to do just that.

Chapter 1: The Uncharted Waters of Parenthood

The day you become a parent, the world shifts beneath your feet. It's a seismic change, a tectonic shift that ripples through every aspect of your life. No amount of reading, no number of well-intentioned friends can truly prepare you for the onslaught of emotions, the weight of responsibility, and the sheer awe that accompanies the birth of a child.

When those first cries echo through the hospital room, it hits you—not just the physical exhaustion, but the profound realization that your life is no longer about you. It's about them—their future, their happiness, their well-being. In that instant, you become their protector, their guide, their everything.

But let me be honest from the start: no one is truly ready to be a parent. And that's okay. Parenting is a journey, not a destination, and there's no roadmap to follow. When my wife and I first embarked on this adventure, we had our fair share of moments where we questioned everything. Were we ready? Could we handle this? We weren't sure we had all the answers, but we knew one thing for certain—we had each other's backs.

Parenting is a partnership, and the moment you're not in lockstep with your spouse or partner, things can unravel quickly.You have to be a team, supporting each other through every high and low. That was one of the most important lessons we learned early on.

We quickly realized that the idea of being "ready" is a bit of a myth. Sure, you can try to prepare. You can stock up on baby gear, read every parenting blog, and try to map out your future as new parents. But when it's 2 AM, and you're rocking a baby back to sleep for the third time that night, all the preparation in the world won't make you feel any more ready. What does make a difference, though, is leaning on the people around you. Your support network—the friends, family, and community that will help you navigate those first days, weeks, and months—is priceless.

Looking back, I realize we probably spent more time "nesting" than we should have. We filled the nursery with all kinds of gadgets and gear that we barely touched. Here's what really mattered: a sturdy crib, a reliable car seat, some diapers, and clothes. The rest? A lot of it came from friends and family who wanted to help. If you're fortunate enough to have that kind of support, lean into it. You don't need to spend a fortune on stuff. What you need is sleep, patience, and help from people who care about you and your new family.

And then there are those first-time experiences. The ones no one can really explain to you until you're in the thick of it.The first time you hear your baby cry—really cry—it pulls at something deep inside you. It's almost primal, this urge to comfort and protect. And in those early days, you'll spend what feels like hours pacing the floors, rocking and soothing a baby who can't yet tell you what they need. Those first cries are just the beginning.

Then comes the first time you hold your baby close and realize that they depend on you for everything. It's both humbling and terrifying. You're responsible for this tiny, vulnerable life, and the weight of that responsibility can be overwhelming.But it's also one of the most rewarding feelings in the world. There's a deep sense of purpose that comes with being a parent, knowing that you are shaping this little person's life.

You'll never forget the first time your baby smiles at you, or the first time they sleep through the night (which, let's be honest, feels like a miracle). Those milestones, while small in the grand scheme of things, feel monumental when they happen. It's those moments that make the sleepless nights and the endless diaper changes worth it. The first time your baby laughs, the first time they reach out for you, the first time they call you "mama" or "dada"—those are the moments that make all the challenges fade away, if only for a little while.

But it's not just the big milestones that matter. There are countless small moments that make up the fabric of parenthood.The quiet moments when you're rocking your baby to sleep, the way they nuzzle into your neck when they're tired, the smell of their skin after a bath—these are the moments that no one prepares you for, but they are the moments that define what it means to be a parent.

The Unpredictable Path

Becoming a parent is like embarking on a journey through uncharted territory. There's no map, no GPS, no clear-cut directions. You're navigating by instinct, by trial and error, and by the occasional stroke of luck.

One day, you'll feel like you've got parenting all figured out. You've got a routine, your baby is sleeping through the night, and you're even managing to get a shower. Then, the next day, everything changes. Your baby starts teething, refuses their usual food, and cries for hours on end. It's like a roller coaster ride, with ups and downs that can leave you feeling dizzy and disoriented.

The key is to remember that this is all part of the process. There will be days when you feel like the best parent in the world, and there will be days when you feel like the worst. It's important to cut yourself some slack and realize that you're doing your best.

The Importance of Self-Care

In the midst of all the chaos and the constant demands of parenthood, it's easy to forget about yourself. But self-care is essential for both your physical and mental well-being. Make time for activities that you enjoy, even if it's just for a few minutes each day. Take a bath, read a book, go for a walk, or simply spend some time alone.

Remember, you can't pour from an empty cup. If you're not taking care of yourself, you won't be able to give your child the love and attention they need.

Conclusion

Becoming a parent is a life-changing experience. It's filled with joy, challenges, and a whole lot of love. There's no right or wrong way to do it. The most important thing is to be present, to be patient, and to love your child unconditionally.

As you embark on this journey, remember that you're not alone. Millions of parents around the world are going through the same thing. Reach out to others for support, share your experiences, and know that you're not alone in this.

Chapter 2: Mom

The role of a mother is hard to put into words, yet it is one of the most defining forces in a child's life. It starts before the child even enters the world, during those nine months when a mother is already nurturing, protecting, and preparing her body and mind for this monumental change. From the moment she holds her baby for the first time, something shifts. It's as though every fiber of her being knows what to do, despite the fact that no one is ever truly prepared for the reality of parenting. A mother is more than just a caretaker. She is the embodiment of safety, security, and unconditional love, a steady presence in her child's life that nothing else can replicate. Her love is instinctive, genetic, and deeply emotional, a force that forms the foundation upon which the rest of a child's life is built.

In our family, my wife plays that role effortlessly. From the very beginning, I could see the connection between her and our children. It wasn't just about meeting their needs or soothing their cries; it was about creating an emotional bond that gave them the confidence to explore the world, knowing they always had a safe place to return to. She was the calming presence when the nights were long and exhausting, and the one who instinctively knew how to comfort them when they were upset. As I watched her, I realized that a mother's love is not something you can fully explain. It's a bond that exists beyond words, something felt on a deeply emotional level by both mother and child.

Mama Bear: The Protector

Every mother I know has something else deep inside her: the "Mama Bear" instinct. It's this primal, protective force that comes out whenever her child is threatened or in need. I've seen it with my wife countless times. When our kids fall and hurt themselves, when they're afraid or upset, or even when someone crosses a line in public, her demeanor shifts. She becomes this fierce protector, and nothing will stand in her way when it comes to ensuring the safety and well-being of our children.

This protective instinct isn't just about physical safety; it's emotional as well. My wife has an almost supernatural ability to know when one of our kids is feeling off, even before they say a word. She can read their emotions, and she knows exactly how to step in to comfort or redirect as needed. It's an incredible skill that seems to come with the territory of being a mom. Whether it's patching up scraped knees, offering words of encouragement, or pulling them into her arms for a hug, she's their constant source of protection.

I remember one day when our youngest was upset about something trivial—something that wouldn't have registered on most people's radar—but to him, it was the end of the world. My wife reached into her bag, pulled out a bandaid, and in that moment, you would've thought she had performed a miracle. The tears stopped, the world righted itself, and all was well again. It wasn't about the bandaid itself. It was about what it represented: comfort, security, and the knowledge that no matter what happens, Mom is always there with a solution, no matter how small.

And then there were the Tic-Tacs. We always had a stash of orange Tic-Tacs on hand, ready to pass off as "medicine" in those moments when only something extra would do the trick. When a child is small, their world is full of bumps, bruises, and imaginary illnesses that need fixing. For them, a bandaid or a Tic Tac could mean everything, and for a mother, it's about knowing when to offer those little comforts to make everything right again.

The Best Mothers I Know

Over the years, I've been fortunate enough to meet and befriend some amazing mothers. They come from all walks of life, each bringing their unique strengths to their roles as parents. Some stay at home, dedicating their entire days to raising their children, while others balance demanding careers with the responsibilities of motherhood. What strikes me about these women is not what they do, but how they do it. The best mothers I know are those who are fully present, who show up for their kids in a way that matters.

One mother I know manages her household like a well-oiled machine. She works full-time but never misses a beat when it comes to her children. Whether it's school plays, bedtime routines, or quiet moments of reassurance, she's always there. She's the mom who manages to balance it all with grace and a sense of humor, never letting the demands of life overshadow her role as a mother. When I see her with her kids, I know they feel loved, valued, and secure. That's what being a good mother is about—not perfection, but presence.

Another friend of ours is a stay-at-home mom, and I've seen her create the most nurturing, warm environment for her children. She's patient, kind, and endlessly creative. Her home is a place where her kids are encouraged to explore, make mistakes, and learn, knowing that their mother is always there to catch them when they fall. She has this way of making her children feel like they are the most important people in the world, and that's a gift not every child receives.

The best mothers I know aren't defined by how much they have or by external achievements. They're defined by the way they make their children feel—safe, loved, and understood. They are there for the big moments and the small ones, offering guidance, support, and a steady presence.

The Worst I've Seen

On the other side of the spectrum, I've also seen mothers who fail to embrace this role. It's not about working or staying home, or even about having tough days (we all have them). It's about the emotional absence, the lack of connection, the mothers who prioritize everything but their children. I've seen mothers who are more concerned with their social media feeds or personal ambitions than with the emotional well-being of their kids. They may provide all the physical necessities—food, clothing, shelter— but the emotional nourishment is nowhere to be found.

Children of these mothers often feel like an afterthought, left to fend for themselves emotionally. They may have the most lavish toys and the best clothes, but they lack the sense of security and love that comes from a mother who is truly present. Watching this is painful because I know the lasting impact it can have on a child. Children need their mothers, not just in a practical sense, but in an emotional, deeply connected way.

Conclusion

Motherhood is one of the most challenging and rewarding roles a woman can take on. It's not about getting everything right, and it's certainly not about being perfect. The best mothers are those who show up for their kids with love, patience, and an unwavering commitment to being there, no matter what. They are the emotional center of their children's lives, the steady force that gives their children the confidence to face the world, knowing they have a safe place to come home to.

In the end, it's not about bandaids, Tic Tacs, or even the Mama Bear instinct—it's about love. A mother's love is one of the most powerful, transformative forces in the world. It's what shapes children into who they are, and it's what stays with them long after they've grown and moved on. Every child deserves that kind of love, and every mother has the power to give it.

Chapter 3: Dad

Fatherhood is often seen through the lens of being a hero. To your child, you're not just a parent; you're their first superhero, the one who makes them feel safe, the one who knows everything, and the one who, in their eyes, can fix anything. Being a dad is about more than just providing; it's about being that constant source of strength, guidance, and love. But the role of a father is complex, shaped by life experiences, both good and bad. It's a journey that requires growth, vulnerability, and a commitment to teaching the values that will shape your child's future.

Hero

In the eyes of a child, their dad is often a larger-than-life figure. For the first few years of their life, you're the one they look up to in awe. It's not about the accolades you've received at work or the number of zeros on your paycheck; to them, you are their hero simply because you're their dad. It's in the way you throw them up in the air and catch them just before they fall, or how you can magically fix a broken toy with a bit of glue and determination. To them, you are invincible, and that belief shapes how they see the world.

For me, the idea of being a hero didn't come naturally. I didn't grow up with a father in the traditional sense, and that left a mark on me in ways I didn't fully understand until I became a dad myself. I didn't have that superhero figure to model myself after, so I had to learn along the way. But the absence of a biological father also gave me a drive to be more, to prove that I could be the dad my kids needed, even if I wasn't sure how to do it at first.

Not Knowing My Biological Father

I didn't know my biological father growing up, and that shaped my understanding of what it meant to be a dad. On one hand, I grew up with a sense of independence, learning to figure things out on my own. But on the other hand, there was always this void, a sense of something missing. I remember being picked on for not knowing sports, for not having that father figure to teach me how to throw a ball or explain the rules of the game. Those moments stung, and they made me feel like I was somehow lacking.

But in a strange way, not knowing my biological father also gave me an incredible sense of determination. It fueled a fire inside me to prove people wrong, to show that I didn't need a traditional father figure to succeed. It gave me the drive to learn on my own, to push myself harder, and to be the best version of myself that I could be. When I became a father, I made a promise to myself that I would be present, that I would be the dad who was there to teach my kids all the things I had to learn on my own.

Not having a father didn't define me, but it did shape the kind of father I wanted to be. It made me more aware of the impact a dad can have, both in his presence and in his absence. And while I didn't have a biological father to look up to, I had strong role models in other areas of my life—teachers, mentors, and family friends—who showed me what it meant to be a man of integrity, to lead with strength and compassion. Those are the lessons I carry with me as a father today.

Protector

One of the most primal instincts as a father is the urge to protect. From the moment your child is born, there's this overwhelming need to shield them from harm, to make sure they're safe at all costs. You become hyper-aware of every potential danger, from the sharp corners of the coffee table to the stranger on the street. You realize that your role is not just to provide, but to protect.

For me, that instinct kicked in the moment I held my child for the first time. It was as if a switch had flipped, and suddenly, I saw the world through a different lens. I became more cautious, more aware of the risks around us, and more determined to keep my family safe. But protection isn't just about physical safety. It's also about emotional safety. As dads, we have a responsibility to protect our children's hearts and minds, to create an environment where they feel secure, loved, and valued.

Being a protector means teaching your children to navigate the world with confidence while knowing they always have a safe place to land. It's about empowering them to take risks, make mistakes, and learn from those experiences, all while knowing that you're there to catch them if they fall. It's a delicate balance between shielding them from harm and allowing them the freedom to grow.

The Strongest Man Alive

For about the first eight years of your child's life, they will think you are the strongest man alive. It doesn't matter if you can't bench press your body weight or if you struggle to open the pickle jar—your kid believes you can do anything. And honestly, it's one of the best feelings in the world.

I leaned into that fantasy with my kids. Whether it was ripping cardboard boxes apart like they were nothing or moving the couch with a dramatic show of strength, I played the role of the "strongest man alive" with pride. I knew those years were limited, and I wanted to give my kids the joy of believing their dad could conquer anything. It wasn't just about showing physical strength, though. It was about giving them a sense of security, letting them know that no matter what happened, Dad was there to handle it.

There's something beautiful about that time in your child's life when they believe in your strength. It's not just about the physical feats you can perform; it's about the strength they see in you as a protector, a provider, and a source of stability. They look to you for guidance, for answers, and for comfort, knowing that in their world, you're the one who keeps everything running smoothly.

Of course, as they get older, they start to realize that you're not actually invincible. They begin to see your flaws and understand that you're human, just like everyone else. But for those precious early years, you get to be their hero, and that's a gift. It's a reminder that fatherhood is about more than just being strong physically; it's about being strong in character, in love, and in commitment.

Authority Figure in Parenting

Being an authority figure as a dad doesn't mean ruling with an iron fist. It's about setting boundaries, creating structure, and teaching your children the value of discipline. Kids need to know that there are rules and consequences, but they also need to know that those rules are rooted in love and a desire to help them grow.

In our house, my wife and I have always emphasized the importance of consistency. Kids thrive when they know what to expect, when they understand the boundaries, and when those boundaries are enforced with fairness and compassion. As a dad, it's my job to make sure that our kids understand the importance of respect—respect for themselves, respect for others, and respect for the world around them.

But being an authority figure also means knowing when to listen, when to be flexible, and when to admit that you don't have all the answers. It's about striking a balance between being firm and being understanding. It's about showing your kids that you're there to guide them, not just to dictate to them. And ultimately, it's about helping them understand that discipline isn't about punishment; it's about learning responsibility and accountability.

Teaching Ethics, Responsibility, and Grit

One of the most important roles of a father is to teach your children the values that will guide them through life. It's not just about telling them right from wrong; it's about modeling it through your actions. Kids are incredibly perceptive. They watch everything you do, and they learn more from what you show them than from what you say.

Teaching ethics starts with showing your kids the importance of honesty, integrity, and kindness. It's about helping them understand that their actions have consequences, not just for themselves but for others as well. It's about instilling in them a sense of empathy and a desire to do the right thing, even when it's hard.

Responsibility is another key lesson. From an early age, we've made it a point to teach our kids that they have a role to play in our family, that their actions matter, and that they are capable of contributing. Whether it's cleaning up their toys, helping set the table, or taking care of their younger siblings, we've always emphasized the importance of responsibility. It's not just about chores; it's about teaching them that they have a part to play in the world, that they are capable of making a difference.

Grit is perhaps one of the most important lessons a father can teach. Life is hard, and there will be challenges along the way. But the ability to persevere, to keep going even when things are tough, is what sets successful people apart. As a dad, I've always tried to teach my kids the value of hard work, resilience, and determination. It's about showing them that failure is not the end—it's just a stepping stone to success.

Chapter 4: Presence is Your Present

As parents, we hear a lot about the importance of being present, but what does that really mean? In today's fast-paced world, where distractions are endless and time feels like a luxury, it's easy to mistake proximity for presence. Having your child sit beside you while you scroll through your phone or watch a movie isn't quite the same as being truly present. The gift of your undivided attention is one of the most precious presents you can offer your child. In the end, your time is how you show your love, and that time needs to be intentional.

Time is Spelled L-O-V-E

If you asked your child what they want most from you, they might not have the words for it, but the answer is simple: time. Time to play, time to talk, time to just be together. They don't care about how much money you make or the size of your house. What matters to them is the time you spend with them. In fact, the way kids spell love isn't L-O-V-E; it's T-I-M-E.

That's why being present isn't just about being physically there. It's about engaging with your child, showing up mentally and emotionally. Sure, sitting together while you watch TV has its moments, and yes, it's great to share the occasional movie night. But if that's the extent of your connection, you're missing out on the deeper, more meaningful interactions that truly build relationships. Watching a movie isn't the same as playing together, asking about their day, or getting on the floor with them to build Legos or color. Those moments of active engagement, of being fully present, are where the real bonding happens.

Reading Books: More Than Just Words

One of the most powerful ways to spend time with your child is through reading. From an early age, we started reading to our kids—bedtime stories, silly books, anything we could find that sparked their imagination. The key to making reading time special was bringing the stories to life. Doing the voices, making them laugh, and diving into the characters turned reading into an experience, not just an obligation.

As they grew older, reading became more than just a fun activity; it became a way to nurture a love for learning and imagination. We made sure that reading wasn't just something they did at school but part of our everyday lives. I set a routine expectation for reading at least 15 minutes a day, not as a chore but as an adventure. And it wasn't just about the words on the page. I'd ask them questions about the plot, the characters, and what they thought would happen next. This wasn't just about ensuring they understood the story; it was about engaging their minds, helping them develop critical thinking, and showing them the joy of getting lost in a book.

Today, my son is a voracious reader, devouring fantasy hero books and comics. He's in the 99th percentile in reading in the nation, and my daughter, a bit younger, is in the 88th percentile. These numbers aren't just about academic achievement; they're a reflection of how a love of reading can unlock doors to creativity, understanding, and confidence. And it all started with being present, with turning storytime into a cherished routine that we built together.

Let Them See You Cry

As dads, we're often taught to be the strong, stoic figure in the family. But one of the most important lessons I've learned is that showing vulnerability doesn't make you weak; it makes you human. Letting your kids see you cry when you're sad or frustrated teaches them that emotions are part of life, and that it's okay to express them.

I've cried in front of my kids, and while those moments felt heavy, they were also important. I remember once when I was going through a particularly rough patch, I broke down in front of them. It wasn't planned, but it happened. Afterward, I made sure to sit with them and explain what I was feeling and how I was working through it. I didn't just leave them with the image of me crying; I followed up to show them that emotions don't last forever, that there's always a way through.

This has created an environment where my kids feel comfortable expressing their own emotions. They don't feel like they have to hide when they're upset or scared. They know it's okay to cry, to talk about their feelings, and to seek comfort when they need it. In showing them my vulnerability, I've given them permission to be vulnerable, too. And that's one of the greatest gifts I can offer them—the knowledge that emotions are normal and that there's strength in working through them together.

Take Them With You to Do Ordinary Things

Sometimes, we think that spending time with our kids requires elaborate outings or special plans. But often, the simplest moments are the ones they remember most. Kids don't need fancy vacations or big events to feel close to you. They just want to be included in your world. Something as simple as taking them with you to the hardware store or letting them tag along on an errand can be a special bonding experience.

I've made it a habit to bring my kids with me whenever I can—whether it's running to the store, getting the car washed, or doing yard work. They love it, not because these activities are exciting, but because they get to be with me. I remember one afternoon when I took my son to the hardware store, and we spent a good half hour just sitting on the tractors in the outdoor section. He was in heaven, not because we bought anything, but because he got to explore and imagine, and I was right there with him, sharing in his excitement.

These ordinary moments build memories. They remind your kids that you don't need a special occasion to spend time together. It's the little things—those quiet, everyday moments—

that truly matter.

Put the Cell Phone Down

In this digital age, it's easy to get distracted. We're constantly bombarded with notifications, emails, and social media. But one of the most important ways to show your child that you're present is to put the phone down. Your child knows when you're not fully engaged, even if you're sitting right next to them. They can sense when your attention is divided, and it sends the message that whatever's on your phone is more important than them.

I'm guilty of it, too. There have been times when I've been in the middle of an email or checking something on my phone, and my child's asked me a question that I only half-heard. But I've learned that when I put the phone down and give them my full attention, the difference is immediate. They light up. They feel seen, heard, and valued. It's a simple action, but it makes a world of difference in building that connection.

How to Be Present With Your Children

Being present is an active choice. It means setting aside distractions and focusing on what matters most—your child. It's about listening, not just hearing. It's about engaging, not just observing. It's about making the most of the time you have, even if that time is limited.

Here are a few ways I've learned to be more present with my kids:

1. Set Boundaries With Work and Technology:
   Make it a point to have tech-free times during the day, especially during meals or family activities. When you're with your kids, be fully with them.

2. Create Rituals:
   Whether it's a bedtime story, a Saturday morning pancake breakfast, or a weekly walk around the neighborhood, create rituals that are just for you and your child. These moments become anchors in their lives, something they can count on and look forward to.

3. Listen With Intent:
   When your child talks to you, put down whatever you're doing and give them your full attention. Ask questions, engage with what they're saying, and show that you care about their thoughts and feelings.

4. Be Consistent:
   Presence isn't just about grand gestures or big

moments; it's about the consistency of being there, day in and day out. Show up, even when it's inconvenient. Be available, even when you're tired. It's the consistency that builds trust and connection.

5. Make Time for One-on-One:
   Whether you have one child or several, it's important to carve out individual time for each of them. These moments allow you to connect on a deeper level and make your child feel uniquely valued.

Ultimately, being present is about making the choice, every day, to show up. To be there, not just in body but in heart and mind. Your time and attention are the greatest gifts you can give your child. In a world full of distractions, being fully present is how you show them that they are truly loved.

Chapter 5: Be Silly, Play

As parents, we often get caught up in the serious side of raising children. We worry about their education, their manners, and their future. But one of the greatest gifts we can give our kids is the ability to be silly, to laugh, and to play. Play isn't just a way to pass the time—it's essential for a child's development and for building the kind of relationship that will last a lifetime.

The Power of Play

Play is a powerful tool for learning, growing, and connecting.
When children play, they aren't just entertaining themselves;
they're exploring the world around them, experimenting with
new ideas, and learning how to navigate emotions and
relationships. Play allows kids to express themselves in ways that
go beyond words. Through play, they learn problem-solving,
empathy, creativity, and resilience.

But perhaps more importantly, play is a way to bond. When you
get down on the floor to build a fort or take part in an epic
pillow fight, you're stepping into their world. You're showing
your child that you care about what makes them happy, that you
value their creativity, and that you're willing to let go of your
adult worries—even if just for a little while—to share in their joy.

Playing together builds trust. It says, "I'm here with you, and I'm
not in a rush to be somewhere else." It fosters a sense of safety
and connection that goes far beyond the games themselves. It's
in those moments of play that you create the memories your
children will carry with them for the rest of their lives.

The Importance of Silliness

There's something magical about being silly with your kids. Silliness breaks down barriers and allows everyone to let go of their inhibitions. Whether it's putting on ridiculous voices during storytime, dancing like no one's watching, or making up silly songs, these moments of unfiltered joy are invaluable.

As adults, we often feel the pressure to be serious, to always have the answers, and to stay in control. But being silly with your children allows them to see another side of you—one that's fun, approachable, and willing to be vulnerable. It shows them that it's okay to laugh at yourself, that life doesn't always have to be taken so seriously.

Silliness is also an important way for kids to develop their sense of humor. Humor is a powerful tool for coping with challenges, building relationships, and finding joy in everyday moments. By being silly with your kids, you're teaching them not only how to laugh but also how to navigate life with a sense of lightness and joy. You're showing them that it's okay to have fun, even in the middle of a busy or stressful day.

Creating a Playful Environment

A playful environment isn't just about having a room full of toys; it's about cultivating an atmosphere where creativity, curiosity, and imagination are encouraged. You can create a playful environment by making room for fun in your daily routines, by being open to spontaneity, and by giving your kids the freedom to explore and imagine.

Start by letting go of perfection. Your house doesn't always have to be spotless, and your schedule doesn't have to be packed with structured activities. Some of the best moments of play happen when there's room for mess, when creativity can flow freely without worrying about rules or outcomes.

Another key to creating a playful environment is encouraging curiosity. Answer your child's endless "why" questions with enthusiasm, and explore the answers together. Foster their imagination by asking them to make up stories, build things with blocks or cardboard, or draw pictures of whatever comes to mind. The goal is to create a space where your child feels safe to express themselves without fear of judgment.

Finally, make time for play. In a world that often prioritizes productivity and achievement, it's easy to see play as a luxury rather than a necessity. But making time for play isn't just important for your kids—it's important for you, too. Playing together strengthens your bond and helps you see the world through your child's eyes. It reminds you to slow down and appreciate the simple joys of life.

Playful Activities

You don't need fancy toys or elaborate plans to engage in playful activities with your kids. In fact, the best games are often the simplest. Here are a few playful activities that encourage creativity, connection, and laughter:

- Imagination Games:
  Whether it's playing pretend, creating imaginary worlds, or taking on different roles, imagination games allow your child to explore new ideas and scenarios. You can turn an ordinary day into an adventure by pretending you're explorers in a jungle or pirates searching for treasure. Let your child take the lead and see where their imagination takes you.

- Build Something Together:
  Whether it's building a fort out of blankets, constructing a LEGO masterpiece, or working on a puzzle, building something together gives you a shared goal. It also teaches patience, problem-solving, and teamwork.

- Silly Competitions:
  Have a dance-off in the living room, make funny faces to see who can hold out the longest without laughing, or challenge each other to a game of charades. These competitions are lighthearted and fun, and they encourage everyone to let loose and enjoy the moment.

- Outdoor Adventures:
  Take your kids to the park, go for a hike, or even just explore your backyard. Nature is the perfect playground, full of opportunities for discovery and play. Whether you're collecting rocks, identifying bugs, or just running around, the outdoors provides endless chances for exploration and fun.

- Storytelling Games:
  Make up stories together, each person adding a sentence or a character to the plot. You'll be amazed at the creative ideas that come up when you collaborate. These storytelling games help develop language skills, creativity, and the ability to think on your feet.

- Crafts and Art Projects:
  Set out some paper, markers, and scissors, and let your child's creativity run wild. Whether you're painting, drawing, or building something out of cardboard, art projects give kids the freedom to express themselves. Plus, the process of creating something together is a great way to bond.

At the end of the day, what matters most isn't what you play or how you play—it's that you take the time to engage with your children in a playful, lighthearted way. Be silly, let go of your adult worries, and enjoy the present moment with your child.

Those moments of play are the foundation of a happy, connected childhood and the memories that will stay with your child for years to come.

Keeping Your House Clean and Teaching Responsibility

As much as play is essential, it's equally important to teach children the value of responsibility. One of the best ways to do that is by involving them in keeping the house clean. Maintaining a tidy home is more than just ensuring things look good; it's about fostering a sense of discipline and ownership in your children. It's also a way to build respect for shared spaces, both within the home and outside of it.

Start with Their Room

A child's room is often their little kingdom, and teaching them to take care of that space is an early lesson in responsibility. Start by giving them small, age-appropriate tasks that they can handle. For younger kids, this might mean putting their toys away or helping you make the bed. As they get older, they can begin to take on more complex tasks, like folding their clothes, vacuuming, or organizing their books and toys.

The goal here isn't to achieve perfection, but to build consistency. Set up a routine where tidying their room becomes a regular part of their day or week. It helps to give them specific guidelines about what "clean" means, like making sure their bed is made, toys are put away, and dirty clothes are in the hamper. By doing this, you're teaching them not just how to clean, but why it's important—to take pride in their space and to understand that keeping things organized is a way of showing respect for themselves and others.

Modeling Cleanliness in Shared Spaces

Children learn best by example. If you're constantly cleaning up after yourself and keeping common areas neat, they're more likely to follow suit. Involve them in family cleaning routines— whether it's wiping down the kitchen counters, sweeping the floor, or organizing the living room. Make it a shared activity, where everyone in the family pitches in. This way, your children will learn that maintaining a clean home is a team effort, not just something that "Mom or Dad does."

Giving your child small responsibilities around the house—like setting the table, feeding the pets, or taking out the trash— teaches them that they are a contributing member of the household. This builds a sense of accomplishment and shows them that their actions matter. They'll start to understand that by completing their tasks, they're helping the entire family function smoothly.

Building Values Through Responsibility

Teaching your children to clean up and care for their belongings is also about instilling core values. When a child understands the importance of keeping their room tidy or helping with household chores, they're learning key principles like responsibility, discipline, and respect. These values go far beyond the walls of your home and will serve them throughout their lives.

1. Responsibility:
   Giving your child tasks around the house shows them that they are responsible for contributing to the family unit. It teaches them that their actions have consequences—whether it's something as simple as feeding the dog on time or making sure their schoolwork is complete. When they take care of their belongings and do their part, they're learning to be accountable for their own actions.

2. Discipline:
   Cleaning their room or completing chores regularly helps children develop self-discipline. It teaches them that not everything in life is fun or easy, but some things need to be done for the greater good. By creating a routine, you're helping your child build the habit of discipline that will extend to other areas of their life, like

schoolwork, relationships, and eventually, their career.

3. Respect:
   Teaching your children to clean up after themselves
   also fosters respect–both for their own things and for
   others. When they learn to care for their belongings,
   they'll be more likely to value what they have and treat
   other people's property with the same care. Respect for
   space and property is a fundamental value that extends
   to relationships with friends, classmates, and eventually
   coworkers.

4. Work Ethic:
   Through regular household tasks, children learn that
   hard work leads to a tangible result–whether that's a
   clean room, a well-set dinner table, or a sparkling
   bathroom. They begin to understand the importance of
   putting in effort to achieve results, a lesson that will
   translate into success in school and their future careers.

Making Clean-Up Fun

Cleaning up doesn't always have to feel like a chore. In fact, you
can turn tidying up into a fun and engaging activity. Use music
as a way to make the process more enjoyable–play their favorite
songs while you clean and turn it into a dance party. You can
also turn it into a game, like setting a timer and seeing how

quickly they can pick up all the toys or giving out "cleaning points" that they can trade for rewards, like extra playtime or a treat.

Another idea is to create a "responsibility chart" where they can track their chores and mark off tasks as they complete them. Visualizing their progress can be incredibly motivating for kids, especially when they can see the results of their hard work.

The Long-Term Impact

When you teach your children to clean up after themselves and contribute to household chores, you're setting them up for long-term success. These small responsibilities prepare them for bigger ones in the future. They'll grow up with a strong work ethic, a sense of personal accountability, and the ability to manage their own time and tasks effectively.

But beyond the practical benefits, involving your children in household responsibilities teaches them the importance of being part of a family, a team, and a community. They learn that they are not just individuals living in their own world, but members of a larger group, each with a role to play in making that group function. And that, ultimately, is one of the most valuable lessons we can pass on to our children.

Chapter 6: "No"

Parenting is often about balance—between love and discipline, freedom and boundaries, yes and no. While saying "yes" feels easier and sometimes more joyful, the power of "no" is where many of the deepest lessons in parenting lie. "No" is more than a simple word; it's a foundation upon which you set boundaries, teach respect, and guide your child toward becoming a responsible adult. But just as important as when parents use "no" is understanding why children use it themselves and how to handle it in ways that promote healthy development.

When a Parent Uses "No"

As parents, we're often the gatekeepers, tasked with keeping our children safe, healthy, and growing into good people. Saying "no" can be uncomfortable, especially when your child is asking for something they really want or when you know it will disappoint them. But "no" is a necessary part of parenting—it's a word that teaches limits, self-control, and the ability to handle disappointment.

When you say "no" as a parent, you're setting boundaries and teaching your child that they can't always have everything they want. This lesson is crucial for their development. Life is full of limits and restrictions, and understanding this early on helps children cope with the inevitable disappointments and frustrations they'll face in adulthood. A parent's "no" is a way of protecting them from harm, be it physical, emotional, or developmental.

For example, saying "no" to an extra cookie before dinner teaches them about self-control and the importance of balanced eating. Saying "no" to staying up late on a school night teaches them responsibility and respect for routine. While it can be hard to be the one who spoils the fun, children actually thrive in environments where boundaries are clear, and "no" is a key part of creating those boundaries.

When a Child Uses "No"

On the flip side, as children grow and begin to assert their independence, "no" becomes one of their favorite words. Any parent of a toddler knows the defiance that can come with this simple, yet powerful word. It can be frustrating to hear your child say "no" to your instructions or rules, but it's important to understand why they use it.

At a developmental level, a child's use of "no" is a sign of growth. It shows that they are beginning to understand their own agency and independence. When a two-year-old shouts "no" at bedtime, they aren't just being defiant—they're testing boundaries and exploring the concept of control. This is a normal part of development, where children begin to realize that they are separate from their parents and can make their own choices.

As they grow older, children use "no" as a way to assert their will. This is a crucial stage in learning self-advocacy. They are learning how to express their preferences, make decisions, and, eventually, stand up for themselves in situations where it matters most. As frustrating as it can be for parents, hearing "no" from your child can be a sign that they are building confidence in their own voice.

The Importance of Boundaries

While "no" is a tool for teaching and asserting independence, it's also a way of establishing boundaries—both for children and parents. Boundaries help children understand where they end and the world begins. They create a sense of security, knowing there are rules and structures they can rely on, even if they don't always like them.

Setting boundaries isn't about being rigid or controlling; it's about teaching your child to respect limits. Whether it's the amount of screen time allowed or the rules about bedtime, boundaries create a framework in which your child can feel safe and understood. Children thrive when they know the rules and can predict the consequences of their actions. They feel secure when they know what is expected of them and what will happen if those expectations aren't met.

Boundaries also help children learn to respect other people's needs and limits. In the long term, this translates into healthier relationships, better emotional regulation, and a more balanced understanding of how to interact with the world around them.

Setting Clear Expectations

One of the best ways to enforce boundaries is by setting clear expectations. Children need to know what is required of them, and these expectations should be communicated in a way they can understand. If expectations are unclear, "no" becomes a constant battle of wills, rather than a learning opportunity.

When setting expectations, it's important to be specific. Instead of saying, "Be good," try something more concrete like, "We don't hit others, and we speak politely." When you give them specific guidelines, you're not only making your expectations clearer, but you're also helping them understand exactly what behavior is expected. This clarity makes it easier for them to follow the rules and feel a sense of accomplishment when they do.

Also, don't be afraid to repeat expectations frequently. Consistency is key in parenting. Children will test boundaries over and over again, so consistent communication is necessary to reinforce those limits.

Consistent Consequences

Consistency is one of the most powerful tools in parenting, especially when it comes to discipline. When you set a boundary and your child crosses it, there should be predictable consequences. This consistency helps children understand that their actions have real outcomes and that the rules aren't arbitrary.

Consequences should be immediate and proportional to the action. For instance, if your child refuses to clean up their toys, the consequence might be that they can't play with them the next day. Or if they hit a sibling, they might need to take a time-out to reflect on their actions. The key is that the consequence should always relate to the behavior in question and be enforced every time the rule is broken.

Inconsistent consequences can be confusing for children. If sometimes they get away with breaking a rule and other times they don't, they may struggle to understand the importance of the boundary. Consistent consequences help to reinforce the lesson that boundaries are meant to be respected, and when they're not, there are real and predictable outcomes.

Positive Reinforcement

While "no" and consequences are essential parts of parenting, so is positive reinforcement. Rewarding good behavior is just as important as correcting bad behavior, if not more so. Children need to know not only what they're doing wrong but also what they're doing right.

Positive reinforcement can come in many forms: praise, rewards, extra playtime, or even just verbal acknowledgment. When your child makes a good choice, follows a rule, or respects a boundary, let them know you noticed. Something as simple as, "I'm really proud of how you shared your toys today," can go a long way in reinforcing positive behavior.

Positive reinforcement helps children understand that their good actions are appreciated and valued. Over time, they'll begin to associate positive feelings with the right choices, making them more likely to repeat those behaviors in the future.

In parenting, the word "no" carries weight. It's a tool to set boundaries, teach important life lessons, and foster independence. But "no" should always be balanced with understanding, communication, and plenty of positive reinforcement. Raising children who respect boundaries while maintaining their self-confidence and sense of independence is a delicate dance, but it's one of the most important tasks of parenthood. In the end, it's not just about saying "no" but about teaching your children why "no" matters, and how it can help them grow into responsible, caring adults.

Giving Them a Chance to Make the Right Choice

As parents, we are often quick to correct our children when they make poor decisions or respond inappropriately. However, there is immense value in giving them a chance to reflect on their behavior and make the right choice on their own. Rather than reacting with anger or frustration when your child says something disrespectful or does something wrong, a simple phrase like,
"I know you know that's not an appropriate answer. Do you want to try that again?"
 can be incredibly effective.

This approach teaches several important lessons. First, it reinforces that you trust your child to know the right behavior, even if they didn't display it the first time. Second, it gives them an opportunity to self-correct without feeling ashamed or attacked. And finally, it shows them that mistakes are not only okay but also opportunities for growth.

For example, if your child speaks to you with an attitude or responds rudely, instead of immediately punishing them or escalating the situation, calmly saying,
"I know you're upset, but I also know you can speak to me more respectfully. Let's try that again,"
 shifts the interaction. You're showing that you expect better from them, but you're also giving them a chance to meet those

expectations on their own terms. The goal here is not to shame them, but to guide them toward better choices.

This method also helps to de-escalate situations. Kids, especially when frustrated or tired, can lash out in ways that they don't necessarily mean. Giving them space to try again allows them to reflect and take responsibility for their actions without feeling like they've already lost the chance to do better. And as parents, it allows us to model patience and forgiveness, showing them that mistakes aren't met with anger, but with understanding and an expectation to improve.

Don't Be Angry—Guide Instead

It's easy to react emotionally when your child does something wrong. After all, parenting is a deeply emotional journey, and when your child pushes boundaries or behaves disrespectfully, it can feel personal. But anger rarely leads to positive outcomes. In fact, when we respond with anger, it can teach our children to either fear us or tune us out.

Instead of reacting with anger, try to guide them with calm and compassion. Remember, children are learning, and every mistake they make is a part of that learning process. When you say,
"I know you know better. Do you want to try again?"
you're not only reinforcing the boundaries but also teaching

them the value of patience and self-reflection.

This approach requires patience, yes, but it also fosters an environment where your child feels safe to admit their mistakes and correct them. They learn that making a wrong choice doesn't define them and that they can always choose to do better next time. This lesson will carry them far beyond childhood, helping them approach life with resilience and a sense of personal responsibility.

By giving them the opportunity to try again and make the right choice, you're teaching your child a critical skill—how to navigate mistakes and handle them gracefully. And in doing so, you're modeling exactly the kind of behavior you want them to carry forward into their own lives.

Chapter 7: "Yes"

As important as it is to say "no," it's equally crucial to know when to say "yes." A parent's "yes" is more than just granting permission—it's about empowering children, encouraging them to explore, and letting them experience life's messes and minor bumps along the way. The word "yes" opens doors, fosters curiosity, and allows your child to feel supported as they navigate the world. In this chapter, we'll explore the power of saying "yes" in parenting, and how it can be a vital tool in raising resilient, confident, and joyful children.

Empowering Children Through "Yes"

Empowerment begins with trust, and trust begins when parents give their children permission to take risks, make decisions, and learn from their experiences. By saying "yes" to new challenges, activities, or responsibilities, we show our children that we believe in their abilities.

Imagine your child asking to try something new—maybe they want to take on a difficult puzzle, bake cookies on their own, or even walk to a friend's house by themselves. These are the moments when a carefully considered "yes" can empower them to believe in their own capabilities. By giving them the green light, you're saying, "I trust you to try, and I trust you to learn."

The flip side of empowerment is, of course, the risk of failure. And that's part of the beauty of saying "yes"—it teaches children how to handle setbacks. When you allow your child to attempt something new, you're giving them the space to experience challenges and find ways to overcome them. Whether they succeed or fail, the real lesson lies in the effort. It's in these moments of "yes" that they learn persistence, creativity, and self-confidence.

Letting Them Be Messy (Or Even A Little Hurt)

One of the hardest parts of parenting is allowing your child to get messy, make mistakes, or even experience a little bit of hurt. Our natural instinct is to protect them from discomfort, but part of growing up is getting dirty—literally and figuratively. Sometimes the best learning happens when they're elbow-deep in mud, or when they fall off a bike and scrape their knee.

Saying "yes" to messy play or activities that might lead to minor scrapes teaches your child resilience. It shows them that life isn't about avoiding every possible risk, but about navigating those risks with care. Sure, letting them splash through a puddle means more laundry, and giving them the freedom to climb a tree might result in a skinned knee. But these small bumps and messes are where they learn to get back up, clean off, and keep going.

There's a powerful lesson in showing your child that it's okay to make a mess or feel a little pain—it's part of the learning process. It's also a chance for you, as a parent, to model how to handle setbacks with grace. When they see you react calmly to a minor injury or help clean up a spill without getting upset, they learn that mistakes and accidents are just part of life, not something to fear or avoid.

The Joy of Saying "Yes"

Saying "yes" can also be a gateway to joy—for both you and your child. In the busyness of life, we can often find ourselves saying "no" out of convenience. It's easier to keep things tidy, predictable, and under control. But what about those moments when "yes" leads to spontaneous fun and connection?

When your child asks you to play a game, build a fort, or go outside in the rain, consider the power of saying "yes." It's in these moments that memories are made, bonds are strengthened, and laughter fills the room. Saying "yes" to fun doesn't mean letting go of all boundaries; it means recognizing the importance of play and the joy that comes with it.

For example, if your child wants to have a pillow fight or set up an elaborate obstacle course in the living room, think about the potential fun and connection it can bring, rather than focusing on the inevitable cleanup. These are the moments your child will remember—the times when you said "yes" to joy, to laughter, to being fully present in their world.

Balancing "Yes" and "No"

Of course, parenting isn't just about saying "yes" all the time. The balance between "yes" and "no" is crucial. Children need structure and boundaries to feel secure, but within those boundaries, "yes" can provide them with the freedom to explore and grow.

As a parent, it's important to discern when "yes" is the right answer. It's not about being permissive or allowing your child to do whatever they want. Rather, it's about thoughtfully considering when to open doors for them. Sometimes, saying "yes" might mean allowing them to try something that feels a little risky, but in a controlled environment. Other times, it might mean granting them independence in areas where they've already shown responsibility.

The key is finding the balance—allowing your child the freedom to make choices and learn from them, while still providing the guidance and safety they need to thrive.

Encouraging Exploration

One of the most powerful uses of "yes" is in encouraging your child to explore the world around them. Whether it's a new hobby, a curious question, or a budding passion, saying "yes" to exploration fosters a sense of wonder and curiosity that will serve them throughout their lives.

If your child shows interest in something new—whether it's science experiments, drawing, building things, or learning about animals—saying "yes" to their curiosity allows them to follow their natural inclinations. These moments of exploration help them discover their strengths and passions, and they teach valuable problem-solving and critical thinking skills.

It's important to remember that exploration doesn't always look neat or organized. It might involve messy kitchens, half-finished projects, or rooms filled with art supplies and science kits. But these are the spaces where creativity and learning thrive. By saying "yes" to exploration, you're giving your child the gift of discovery and the confidence to pursue what excites them.

Building Self-Reliance Through "Yes"

Another crucial aspect of saying "yes" is fostering self-reliance. When you allow your child to take on responsibilities and make decisions, you're helping them build the skills they need to become independent. This can be as simple as letting them choose their own clothes for the day, make their own breakfast, or plan a family outing. While these decisions may seem small, they're actually significant opportunities for your child to practice autonomy and feel capable.

When your child asks if they can try something new, respond with a thoughtful "yes" whenever it's safe and reasonable.

Maybe it's cooking dinner for the family, handling their homework without reminders, or navigating a social situation on their own. These moments of empowerment teach them that they can trust themselves to take on challenges and find solutions.

Over time, this builds resilience and confidence—traits that will serve them well throughout their lives. The more you say "yes" to their abilities, the more they'll come to believe in themselves and their capacity to handle whatever comes their way.

In a world filled with rules, boundaries, and expectations, "yes" can be a powerful tool in raising confident, capable, and joyful children. It empowers them to take risks, make choices, and learn from their experiences. It shows them that life is meant to be explored, even if that means getting a little messy or encountering a few bumps along the way. And most importantly, it teaches them that they are trusted, valued, and supported as they grow into the best versions of themselves.

Chapter 8: Social Skill Building

Raising children to be socially competent and emotionally intelligent is a crucial part of parenting. The ability to navigate social interactions, handle conflicts, and engage confidently with the world doesn't come naturally to everyone—it's something that must be nurtured and practiced. As parents, we play a key role in shaping our children's social skills, helping them learn how to interact with others in meaningful and respectful ways. In this chapter, we'll explore how simple everyday actions, challenges, and activities can contribute to building these essential skills.

Take Them with You to Do Normal Things

One of the best ways to teach social skills is through exposure to real-life situations. Taking your child with you as you go about your daily routines—grocery shopping, running errands, visiting the bank—gives them the opportunity to observe and engage in everyday social interactions. These outings become valuable teaching moments, showing them how to talk to people, ask for help, and even handle minor frustrations.

Children are naturally curious about the world around them, and involving them in the normal tasks of life helps demystify the social norms they'll encounter as they grow. When they see you greet the cashier, ask questions, or handle small conflicts with patience and kindness, they learn by watching you. You're modeling behavior in real time.

But don't just let them observe—encourage participation. Have your child ask the clerk where to find an item in the store or hand money to the cashier. This builds confidence and helps them practice communication in low-pressure situations. It also teaches them that they are a part of the family unit, with responsibilities and contributions to make, no matter how small.

Let Them Do Hard Things

Social skill building is not just about being polite or making friends. It's also about developing resilience, grit, and the ability to handle adversity. One of the most valuable lessons we can give our children is the opportunity to do hard things. Whether it's facing a challenge at school, working through a difficult problem, or navigating a tricky social situation, the ability to persevere is key to functioning in society.

Letting your children face hard things can be difficult as a parent. Our instinct is to step in and protect them from struggle, but it's in those moments of challenge that real growth happens. When they have the opportunity to tackle something difficult—whether it's standing up for themselves in a social setting or completing a tough project—they learn how to manage stress, work through frustration, and find solutions.

For example, if your child is struggling with a school assignment, resist the urge to give them the answers. Instead, guide them through the problem-solving process. Encourage them to keep trying, remind them that it's okay to make mistakes, and praise their efforts, not just their results. By doing this, you're teaching them the value of persistence and the satisfaction of overcoming obstacles, which are both essential social skills in adulthood.

Sports and How They Can Help

Team sports are one of the most effective ways to help children learn how to function as part of a community. Whether it's soccer, basketball, or baseball, participating in sports teaches children how to cooperate, communicate, and handle both victory and defeat with grace.

Sports instill the value of teamwork. On the field or court, children quickly learn that individual efforts are important, but success often depends on how well they work with others. This is a critical social lesson—learning to collaborate with different personalities, compromise, and work toward a common goal.

Additionally, sports provide structured opportunities for children to handle conflict. There will be moments when they disagree with a teammate, feel frustrated with their own performance, or experience disappointment in losing a game. These are all opportunities to develop emotional regulation and conflict resolution skills. As parents, it's our job to guide them through these moments, helping them process their feelings and teaching them how to communicate effectively with their peers.

Furthermore, sports can foster a sense of responsibility. Whether it's showing up for practice, following the rules, or being accountable for their role on the team, children learn that their actions have consequences. This accountability is essential for functioning well in any social setting, as it teaches children to be dependable and considerate of others.

How to Handle Conflict with Others

Conflict is a natural part of life, and it's inevitable that your child will experience it in various forms—whether with siblings, friends, or even you as a parent. Teaching children how to handle conflict constructively is one of the most important social skills they can learn.

When conflict arises, it's crucial to model calm and respectful communication. Children are often emotionally driven, especially when they feel wronged or frustrated, and it's our role as parents to guide them through the process of resolving disagreements in a healthy way. Instead of jumping to conclusions or immediately intervening, encourage your child to explain their perspective and listen to the other person's side.

For example, if there's a disagreement between siblings, ask each child to take turns sharing how they feel, without interruption. This practice of active listening not only helps resolve the current issue but also teaches empathy—an essential skill for forming and maintaining healthy relationships.

Another useful tool in conflict resolution is helping your child reframe situations. Instead of seeing every disagreement as a battle to be won, guide them toward solutions where both parties can feel heard and satisfied. This shift in mindset—from competition to cooperation—builds emotional intelligence and sets the foundation for more positive interactions in the future.

Handling Conflict with You

Conflict with parents is inevitable, especially as children grow and test boundaries. How you handle these moments can shape their understanding of authority and respect for others.

One effective strategy is to give your child the opportunity to correct themselves. Instead of reacting with immediate frustration when they push back or give an inappropriate response, say something like, "I know you know that's not an appropriate answer. Do you want to try that again?" This gives them a chance to reflect, correct their behavior, and make the right choice—without feeling shamed or scolded.

This method not only teaches self-regulation but also reinforces the idea that mistakes are opportunities for learning, not occasions for punishment. It shifts the focus from controlling behavior to encouraging responsibility, which is a far more effective approach in the long term.

Ordering Food: A Step Toward Independence

One of the simplest but most powerful ways to build social skills and foster independence is by encouraging your child to order their own food at restaurants. It might seem like a small thing, but the act of speaking up, making a choice, and interacting with a server is a big step in their social development.

When your child orders their own food, they're practicing communication, decision-making, and assertiveness. It's a chance for them to articulate what they want, engage in a polite conversation, and feel a sense of independence. Even if they're shy at first, the more they practice, the more confident they'll become in expressing themselves in social situations.

This simple act also reinforces the idea that they are capable individuals who can advocate for themselves. It's a step toward autonomy, showing them that they don't need you to manage every interaction for them—they can handle things on their own, even in small ways.

Building Responsibility Through Social Interaction

Social skills and responsibility go hand in hand. When children learn how to interact with others respectfully, they also learn the importance of being responsible for their actions and words.

Whether it's taking ownership of a mistake, fulfilling a promise, or simply being kind and considerate, these lessons extend beyond social interactions and into every aspect of life.

One way to build responsibility is by giving your child opportunities to contribute to the family in meaningful ways. This might mean assigning them chores, asking for their help with tasks around the house, or giving them responsibilities like taking care of a pet. These tasks not only teach practical life skills but also instill a sense of accountability and the understanding that they are part of a larger community—their family.

When children see that their contributions matter, they begin to understand the value of responsibility and how it plays a crucial role in their relationships with others. This sense of accountability, coupled with strong social skills, will serve them well as they navigate friendships, school, and eventually, the workplace.

Social skill building is an ongoing process, one that requires patience, practice, and plenty of real-world experience. By involving your child in everyday activities, allowing them to face challenges, encouraging participation in team sports, and guiding them through conflicts, you're giving them the tools they need to thrive socially. These skills not only help them navigate relationships and interactions today but also set the foundation for their future success as adults.

Chapter 9: The Choice Method

If there is one parenting tip I would share above all others, it's the power of the
Choice Method
. This simple yet profound approach can transform your relationship with your children, especially in those younger years when power struggles seem to dominate daily life. The Choice Method offers children the illusion of control, while you, as the parent, still guide the outcome. You can call it what you

want—"structured freedom" or "guided independence"—but this method will save you from countless battles, tantrums, and tears.

At its core, the Choice Method works because of its grounding in developmental psychology. Young children are driven by a strong need for autonomy and control as they begin to explore the world around them. When you give them choices within boundaries that you set, you empower them to feel like they have control over their decisions, which reduces defiance and increases cooperation. The key is to create choices that you, as the parent, are equally comfortable with. It's about giving options that serve your needs, while allowing your child to feel involved and capable.

The Psychology Behind the Choice Method

The developmental psychology that underpins this method relates to a child's evolving sense of autonomy. Around age two, children begin to assert their independence as they move from complete dependence on caregivers to wanting to do things themselves. This is where the classic phrase "the terrible twos" comes in, often fueled by power struggles between what the parent wants and what the child wants. This stage is a critical period for building the foundation of a child's self-efficacy, or their belief in their ability to influence the world around them.

From a psychological standpoint, when children feel they have some control, they are less likely to resist, throw tantrums, or act out. Research in developmental psychology shows that offering choices can reduce oppositional behavior because it respects a child's growing desire for autonomy while still providing structure and boundaries.

Erik Erikson's stages of psychosocial development
 include the phase of "autonomy vs. shame and doubt," where toddlers begin to seek independence. If children are overly controlled or not given the opportunity to assert their will, they may develop doubt in their own abilities, leading to a lack of confidence. The Choice Method taps into this developmental need, giving children an age-appropriate sense of control that fosters independence and confidence while reducing frustration for both parent and child.

5 Examples of How Situations Are Typically Handled vs. the Choice Method

Let's break this down with practical, real-world examples. Here are five common parenting scenarios and how applying the Choice Method could radically shift the dynamic.

Example 1: Mealtime Battles

Typical Approach
: You serve dinner, and your child refuses to eat vegetables. You demand they eat them, which turns into a standoff. They refuse more aggressively, and you threaten consequences if they don't eat. Now, the focus is on the battle, not the food.

The Choice Method
: Instead of presenting the meal as a non-negotiable, offer a simple choice: "Would you like broccoli or carrots with dinner?" Either option is a win for you, and they feel empowered because they got to choose. You've transformed the situation from a power struggle into a decision-making process.

Example 2: Getting Dressed

Typical Approach
: It's time to get dressed, and your child wants to wear pajamas to school. You say no, they insist. You argue back and forth, and the morning quickly devolves into a meltdown.

The Choice Method
: Present your child with two acceptable clothing options: "Do you want to wear the red shirt or the blue shirt today?" This provides them with autonomy within boundaries you've already set. They still feel like they're making the decision, but the battle over pajamas never begins because you've preemptively

framed the choices in a way that avoids conflict.

Example 3: Bedtime Routine

Typical Approach
: It's bedtime, but your child doesn't want to go to bed. You tell them it's time, they resist, and it turns into a drawn-out negotiation, or worse, a tantrum. Everyone ends up frustrated.

The Choice Method
: Before bedtime, offer two choices: "Would you like to read one book or two before bed?" Or, "Do you want to brush your teeth first or put on your pajamas first?" By giving them agency over the routine, they're more likely to comply without resistance. The choice empowers them, but you still achieve the goal of getting them to bed.

Example 4: Leaving the Playground

Typical Approach
: Your child doesn't want to leave the playground. You tell them it's time to go, and they cry or throw a tantrum, refusing to leave. You're stuck between dragging them away or standing there negotiating.

The Choice Method
: Before it's time to leave, say, "We're leaving in five minutes. Do you want to go down the slide one more time or swing one more time before we go?" This preemptive choice gives them a sense of control over the transition. They still have to leave, but they feel like they got to decide how to end their time at the playground.

Example 5: Homework Time

Typical Approach
: You tell your child it's time to do homework, and they resist, saying they don't want to do it now. You push back, and it turns into a battle of wills, with each side growing more entrenched.

The Choice Method
: Instead of dictating when homework starts, offer a choice: "Do you want to do your homework now and play later, or play for 10 minutes and then do homework?" Both choices lead to the same outcome, but your child feels like they have a say in when and how they tackle the task. You've reduced resistance by giving them a sense of control.

The Illusion of Control

At the heart of the Choice Method is the concept of the illusion of control. Children crave autonomy, but they also need structure. By giving them choices within limits, you meet their psychological need for independence while maintaining parental guidance. The magic of the Choice Method is that it gives children a sense of control, even though you are the one setting the parameters.

It's important to note that the choices you present should always be ones that you, as the parent, are comfortable with. Never offer a choice that you aren't willing to follow through on. For example, if you give your child the option to stay at the playground for 10 more minutes or leave immediately, be prepared to honor whichever choice they make.

This approach not only helps avoid power struggles, but it also teaches your child decision-making skills. They begin to understand the consequences of their choices and learn how to weigh options—valuable skills that will serve them well throughout life.

The Power of Saying "Yes"

An essential part of the Choice Method is the ability to say "yes" more often. By presenting choices, you are effectively saying "yes" to your child's input, while still guiding their behavior in the direction you need it to go. This positive reinforcement fosters cooperation, encourages open communication, and reduces the tension that comes with constant commands and refusals.

When children hear "no" too often, they can become frustrated, resentful, and more likely to rebel. The Choice Method flips this script by empowering them with the opportunity to make choices, leading to a more harmonious dynamic.

Conclusion

The Choice Method is one of the simplest yet most effective tools in a parent's arsenal. It respects a child's need for autonomy, helps them develop decision-making skills, and reduces power struggles that can strain the parent-child relationship. By offering choices within boundaries, you give your child a sense of control while still guiding them toward positive outcomes. Whether it's mealtime, bedtime, or any other daily task, the Choice Method turns potential conflict into an opportunity for growth and cooperation.

Chapter 10: The Big Struggle

Parenting often feels like a tightrope walk. On one side, you want to give your children the freedom to learn, grow, and explore the world around them. On the other, you have the primal instinct to protect them from harm, shield them from adversity, and keep them safe. Balancing freedom, learning, safety, autonomy, and creating the drive they'll need to succeed —it's not just hard; it can feel impossible at times.

And the truth is, it is impossible to get it right 100% of the time. There's no perfect formula. You may feel like you're heading down a path blindly, unsure if the choices you're making are the right ones. But here's something I've learned: feeling that way is not a sign of failure. It's normal. Every parent has felt that uncertainty, that push-and-pull between giving too much or too little. The key to navigating this journey is a blend of knowledge, experience, and deep understanding of your child.

Let's dive into the elements of this delicate balancing act.

Freedom vs. Safety

When you first become a parent, the thought of your child getting hurt can feel unbearable. From baby gates to helmets, our instinct is to wrap them in bubble wrap and keep them out of harm's way. But as they grow, you start to realize that preventing every fall or scrape is not only impossible but also unwise. Kids need to get hurt occasionally—physically, emotionally, socially—to learn how to handle life's inevitable bumps and bruises.

Freedom and safety are in constant tension. Too much freedom, and your child might find themselves in danger. Too much safety, and they might never learn how to handle the world on their own. So how do you balance this?

For me, it's been about calculated risks. When my kids want to climb higher than I think is safe, I don't immediately tell them no. Instead, I'll spot them, ready to catch them if necessary, but allowing them the space to challenge their limits. You can't—and shouldn't—control everything, but you can be there to guide them through the tough moments.

Autonomy vs. Control

One of the biggest struggles in parenting is knowing when to let go. It starts when they're toddlers—letting them dress themselves, even if it means mismatched clothes and shoes on the wrong feet. It continues through their teen years—letting them make decisions that you may not agree with but that are essential for their growth.

It's hard to give them autonomy because, as a parent, you naturally want to control things. You think, "I know best. I can save them from mistakes." But here's the thing: autonomy builds resilience. Kids need to make mistakes to learn from them.

The key is offering choices that allow them to practice autonomy while keeping within safe boundaries. Remember the "choice method" we discussed earlier? It applies here, too. By offering choices, you're empowering them to take control of their lives in small, manageable ways. These little decisions add up and help them learn responsibility without feeling stifled by your rules.

Adversity Leads to Growth

No one wants their child to suffer, but adversity is a powerful teacher. When we shield our children from every challenge, we rob them of the opportunity to develop grit, perseverance, and problem-solving skills.

It's tough to watch your child struggle—whether it's a tough class, a difficult social situation, or a hard loss in a sport. But those struggles are essential. I've seen it in my own kids. When they face something hard, I want to rush in and fix it. But I've learned to hold back. I offer support and encouragement, but I don't always intervene. Watching them overcome challenges— seeing that lightbulb moment when they realize they can do it— has been some of the most rewarding moments of my parenting journey.

It's not about throwing your kids into the deep end. It's about giving them opportunities to face adversity in a way that's developmentally appropriate and supportive. Let them fall, but be there to help them back up.

Building Self-Esteem

Self-esteem is not built by constantly praising your child for every little thing they do. It's built by allowing them to struggle, overcome, and achieve. It's built by letting them solve problems on their own and learn from their mistakes.

Too often, we think that protecting our kids from failure will boost their self-esteem, but the opposite is true. Kids who never face failure often grow up to be adults who crumble at the first sign of adversity. Let your kids know that failure is not something to be feared—it's part of the learning process.

Celebrate their efforts more than their outcomes. Praise the hard work, not just the result. This helps your child understand that success is a journey, not a destination.

Good Friends, Bad Friends

As your children grow, their social circles will expand, and with that comes the challenge of navigating friendships. Not every friend will be a good influence, and it's inevitable that your child will cross paths with kids who don't share the same values you're trying to instill at home.

The instinct to control who your child hangs out with is strong, but banning certain friends outright can backfire. Instead, focus on teaching your child how to recognize good and bad behaviors in friendships. Encourage open conversations about their relationships. Ask them how they feel after spending time with certain friends. Do they feel uplifted or drained? Happy or stressed? Teach them to listen to those cues.

Good friends help build self-esteem and resilience; bad friends can undermine those same qualities. Helping your child learn to choose their friendships wisely is far more powerful than dictating who they can or cannot spend time with.

Good Parents, Bad Parents

No parent is perfect. We all have moments where we question ourselves or where we feel like we've made the wrong call. And that's okay. What matters is that we keep striving to be better, to learn from our mistakes, and to adapt as our children grow.

One of the most important things I've learned is to never compare myself to other parents. There will always be parents who seem to have it all together—whose kids seem perfectly well-behaved, who seem to handle every situation with grace. But you don't know what's happening behind closed doors. Every family has its struggles, and every parent has their moments of doubt.

At the same time, I've learned a lot from observing other parents—both the good and the bad. I've seen parents who are overly controlling and whose kids rebel because of it. I've seen parents who are too lax, whose kids have no boundaries or sense of responsibility. I've tried to take the best lessons from the parents I admire and learn from the mistakes I've seen others make.

Finding Balance

Balancing all of these elements—freedom, safety, autonomy, control, adversity, self-esteem—is a lifelong struggle. You're not always going to get it right, and that's okay. Parenting is about learning and adapting as you go.

One of the best tools I've found is combining research with my own experience. Read about parenting techniques, talk to other parents, and most importantly, get to know your child. Every child is different, and what works for one might not work for another. Tailor your approach to fit your child's personality, strengths, and needs.

At the end of the day, there's no one-size-fits-all approach to parenting. The best you can do is keep learning, stay present, and trust that you are doing the best you can.

Chapter 11: The Guiding Principle

One of the core principles I've tried to live by as a parent is simple: you want your kids to run
to
 you, not
from
 you. This is not just about avoiding punishment or keeping secrets—it's about fostering a deep sense of trust, safety, and openness that allows your children to feel comfortable coming to you, no matter the situation. This principle has guided nearly every decision I've made as a father, from discipline to how I

spend my time with my kids.

The heart of this idea is trust. When your child trusts you–when they know you'll listen, that you won't overreact, and that you have their back–they'll come to you when it matters most. That doesn't mean there won't be rules or consequences. It means that discipline, trust, and self-esteem must always be in balance, creating a home environment where mistakes are opportunities for growth, not fear.

Trust

Trust is the foundation of every strong relationship, and parenting is no different. But trust doesn't come automatically–it has to be earned over time. It's built in those little moments when your child feels heard, understood, and respected. Trust grows when your child knows that, even in moments of frustration or disappointment, your love for them is unwavering.

In practical terms, trust means giving your child the benefit of the doubt. It means believing in their intentions, even when their actions don't always align. It means showing them that, while you may not always agree with their choices, you will always be there to help them figure things out.

But trust is also a two-way street. Just as you want your child to trust you, it's important to show them that you trust them. This doesn't mean blind trust, but rather giving them responsibilities and freedoms that demonstrate your belief in their ability to make good choices. This could be as simple as trusting them to take on a task independently or as significant as trusting them to navigate a difficult social situation on their own.

When your children feel trusted, they will rise to meet that trust. They'll work harder to make good decisions, not just to avoid punishment, but because they don't want to let you down. And when they stumble—as they inevitably will—they'll come to you for help instead of hiding it, because they know that trust means they won't be met with anger or shame, but with guidance and understanding.

Balancing Discipline, Trust, and Self-Esteem

Discipline is necessary. It's how children learn boundaries, right from wrong, and the consequences of their actions. But discipline should never erode trust or self-esteem. The goal of discipline should be to teach, not to punish.

When discipline is rooted in anger, frustration, or disappointment, it can damage the very trust we're trying to build. This is where balance comes in. The most effective discipline comes from a place of love and respect. It's not about wielding power or authority over your child; it's about helping them understand why certain behaviors are unacceptable and guiding them toward better choices.

One way to maintain this balance is by offering second chances. When a child makes a mistake, instead of immediately jumping to punishment, try saying, "I know you know that's not an appropriate answer. Do you want to try that again?" This gives them the opportunity to correct their behavior on their own, fostering responsibility while maintaining their dignity. It also shows them that you believe they are capable of making the right choice, which builds both trust and self-esteem.

Another important aspect is ensuring that consequences are consistent, but not overly harsh. The goal is to help your child understand the impact of their actions, not to make them feel bad about themselves. If consequences are too extreme, your child might start to fear you rather than trust you, and that's when they'll begin to run from you instead of to you.

The Importance of Spending Time Together

There's no shortcut to building trust and maintaining balance in your parenting. It takes time, attention, and consistency. And that time is most critical when your children are young. The earlier you invest in building strong, trusting relationships with your kids, the more resilient those bonds will be as they grow.

Research backs this up. Studies consistently show that spending quality time with your children when they are young has a profound impact on their development. Children who regularly spend time with their parents tend to have higher self-esteem, better emotional regulation, and stronger social skills. They're also more likely to come to their parents with their problems, rather than hiding them.

A study published in the
Journal of Family Psychology
found that parental involvement, particularly in early childhood, was linked to higher academic achievement, fewer behavioral problems, and stronger emotional health later in life. Another study from the
Harvard Graduate School of Education
highlighted that children who feel close to their parents are more likely to make responsible decisions in adolescence and beyond. The message is clear: time spent with your children is one of the best investments you can make in their future.

The Power of Running
To
You: Examples

Let's imagine a scenario that plays out in homes every day: something breaks. Maybe it's a vase, a toy, or—if you're really unlucky—a screen. Your child, wide-eyed and anxious, looks at you, waiting for the inevitable fallout. In many homes, this is a moment of fear. The child knows that yelling, anger, and punishment are on the way. So, they might try to hide it, lie about it, or blame someone else.

But what if your child knew they could come to you instead? What if, even though they're scared, they trusted you enough to tell you what happened, knowing you'd respond with understanding first, before addressing the consequences? In this scenario, they would say, "Mom, Dad, I broke this, and I'm really sorry." You'd still need to talk about how to be more careful in the future, and there may still be consequences like helping to pay for the damage or losing screen time, but the initial response wouldn't be about punishment. It would be about problem-solving together. And that's what builds trust.

Now take that same concept and apply it to a more serious scenario: your child is a teenager, and they're at a party. They know they're not supposed to be drinking, but peer pressure kicks in, and they've had a drink or two. It's late, and they realize they don't want to drive or stay there. In that moment, many teens would hesitate to call their parents, fearing the backlash.

But if you've built that relationship of trust—if your child knows that they can come to you, even in a moment of poor decision-making—they'll pick up the phone. They'll call you because they trust that, while there may be consequences, you won't react with anger first. You'll pick them up, ensure they're safe, and have the important conversation about choices and responsibility later.

That's the power of the guiding principle: creating an environment where your children trust you enough to come to you, no matter the circumstances.

The Long Game

Parenting is not about being perfect, and it's certainly not about having all the answers. It's about being there, consistently, day after day, showing your children that no matter what happens, you will always love them, you will always guide them, and they can always trust you.

This guiding principle of trust—ensuring that your children run to you rather than from you—ties directly into earlier chapters, reinforcing key lessons about presence, discipline, and empowerment. In Chapter 4, we talked about how "presence is your present," and it's this consistent presence that lays the foundation for trust. By being there for the ordinary moments and showing vulnerability, you create an emotional safety net that encourages your child to come to you in times of need. Similarly, in Chapter 6, when we discussed the importance of boundaries and saying "no," we emphasized that discipline, when handled thoughtfully, builds trust rather than fear. And in Chapter 7, "Yes," we explored how empowering children to take risks–letting them be messy or even get hurt–teaches them responsibility. The guiding principle pulls these ideas together, showing that trust isn't built in isolated moments, but through a balance of presence, boundaries, and empowerment, forming the bedrock of your relationship with your child.

The goal is not to raise children who never make mistakes. The goal is to raise children who, when they do make mistakes, know that they can turn to you for help. By balancing discipline, trust, and self-esteem, you're creating the foundation for a relationship that will last well beyond their childhood years. You're showing them that, no matter how big or small the problem, they can always run to you.

Chapter 12: Aligning with Your Partner

If you are fortunate enough to be navigating parenthood with a partner, the most important foundation is staying aligned with one another. The role of two parents is a powerful tool, but it only works when both are pulling in the same direction. Kids are incredibly perceptive; they quickly pick up on inconsistencies between parents, and if you're not careful, they will learn to exploit those gaps. The key is to stay connected and approach parenting as a team with shared goals and consistent boundaries.

The aim is simple: make things easier for one another. Parenting is hard enough without unintentionally undermining each other. Being in lock step with your partner means not only agreeing on the big-picture goals for your kids but also supporting each other in the daily grind of decision-making.

My wife and I have regular check-ins. We make time—sometimes daily, sometimes weekly—to discuss what's been going on with the kids. We talk about their behavior, what we're each addressing, and where we might need help from the other. This not only keeps us aligned but also ensures we're not duplicating efforts or contradicting one another.

It's important to acknowledge that children will behave differently with each parent. For example, our youngest has learned that my wife tends to be more nurturing and protective, often avoiding hurt feelings at all costs. That instinct is beautiful, and part of what makes her an amazing mom, but it can lead to situations where the kids learn to manipulate a bit. One recent example was when our youngest didn't eat lunch but managed to sneak in some iPad time instead. My wife, out of a desire to avoid conflict, let it slide. That's where I stepped in. I enforced the consequences we had both agreed on—no screen time until meals are eaten—and afterward, I provided her with supportive feedback. It wasn't a criticism, just a moment to realign our parenting so we're sending a consistent message to our child.

The key here is communication. You both need to be on the same page when it comes to discipline, reward systems, and general expectations. When we're consistent, our kids feel safe—they know what to expect and aren't confused by mixed messages. But consistency also requires support. We each have moments of weakness, and that's okay. It's when you have a partner who can pick up the slack in those moments that the team effort shines.

At the end of the day, it's about balance. I tend to be more authoritative when it comes to enforcing rules, while my wife leans into the nurturing side. That combination is powerful if managed well, but it requires constant attention and effort. We regularly remind each other that we're in this together, always with the same goal: to raise confident, respectful, and well-adjusted kids.

Chapter 13: Your Community of Parents

Raising children isn't something you do in isolation—it truly takes a village. Your community of parents plays a critical role in shaping your journey, offering support, advice, and often, a much-needed sense of camaraderie. It's easy to feel alone in the chaos of parenthood, but knowing you have others who are walking the same path can make all the difference.

For us, our community started with other parents at school, daycare, and even the park. There's something instantly bonding about sharing parenting war stories, trading tips, or simply venting about the sleepless nights and tantrums. These moments are invaluable because they remind you that you're not alone.

When you're connected to other parents, you gain different perspectives on how to handle various situations. I've lost count of how many times I've taken advice from another dad on how to handle a tough discipline situation, or when my wife has gotten tips from other moms on navigating sibling rivalry. You don't always have to follow the advice to the letter, but hearing how other people manage their challenges can spark ideas that help you refine your own parenting approach.

But the benefits of a parent community go beyond advice. It's about creating a support system. Whether it's carpooling to soccer practice or hosting a sleepover, having other families you can rely on lightens the load. My wife and I have been fortunate to have a tight-knit group of parent friends who we trust completely. If one of us is running late or needs an extra hand, we know someone in our circle will step in. And that reciprocity builds deeper relationships not just among the adults but also among the kids.

There's also an element of accountability that comes with being part of a parent community. When you see how others are handling similar situations, it can challenge you to reflect on your own choices. It might push you to be more patient, more creative, or more disciplined. Parenting isn't a competitive sport, but we can learn a lot from observing each other.

At the end of the day, building a community of parents isn't just about practical support. It's about creating a network where your kids can see the value of relationships, collaboration, and shared experiences. When your children see you building these connections, they learn the importance of community and the value of leaning on others.

Sometimes it's the simplest moments that bring it home—like a group BBQ where the kids run wild while the adults laugh over the fire, or the after-school debrief with a fellow parent about a school project. These shared moments shape our children just as much as they shape us as parents.

So, if you don't have a parent community yet, I encourage you to find one. Reach out at school events, sign your kids up for group activities, or even start conversations at the playground. The friendships you build can provide strength, guidance, and connection as you navigate the ups and downs of raising children.

Story 1: A Friend Asking for Help

One evening, I got a call from a close friend. I could hear the anxiety in his voice before he even spoke. "I need to talk to you about something," he said, hesitating for a moment. "I just found out my son is gay."

There was a pause, the weight of his words hanging in the air. I could tell he was trying to process it all—his expectations, his fears, and, most of all, how to respond in a way that would support his child. He wasn't angry, just unsure of how to handle something that had never crossed his mind.

We met up that night, and as we sat together, he opened up about his feelings. "It's not that I don't love him or support him," he said. "I just don't know how to navigate this. I wasn't prepared for it, and I'm worried about what his life will be like. How do I protect him?"

I listened, understanding the complexity of his emotions. The first thing I told him was that he didn't need to have all the answers immediately. "What your son needs most right now is to know that you're in his corner. You don't need to fix anything or say all the right things. Just let him know you love him, and that you'll be there no matter what."

We talked about how difficult this moment must have been for his son, to share something so personal, likely with fear of judgment or rejection. I reassured him that the fact his son had the courage to come to him was a sign of deep trust. I reminded him that being there, being present, and continuing to nurture that trust was the most important thing he could do.

I also shared that, as parents, we're always learning, always adjusting. Sometimes we don't feel ready for the curveballs, but what matters is how we show up. And in this case, it was about showing unconditional love, not just in words but in action. He left that conversation with a little more clarity, knowing that even if he felt uncertain, he was doing the right thing by being there for his son.

Story 2: Me Asking for Help

A few months ago, I found myself in a situation where I had to ask for help, and it wasn't easy for me. My son had been struggling in baseball, specifically with fielding in the outfield. No matter how much we practiced, whenever the ball came to him, he would freeze. He wanted so badly to get it right, but his frustration mounted with every missed catch. He was losing confidence, and I was feeling helpless.

I've always prided myself on being able to teach my kids resilience, to push through challenges. But in this case, no matter how much I encouraged him, he couldn't get past the mental block. I felt stuck and knew that if I kept pushing without figuring out a new approach, it might do more harm than good.

So, I reached out to another dad from our baseball league, someone whose son was also on the team and had faced similar struggles. This wasn't easy for me—I'm used to being the one offering advice, not asking for it. But I realized that if I wanted to help my son, I needed to be open to new ideas.

I explained the situation, and this dad didn't judge. Instead, he shared some insight from his own experience. "Have you tried breaking it down into smaller steps?" he asked. "Sometimes it's not about the physical skill, but the mental pressure they're feeling. Start with something smaller, easier to catch—like a tennis ball. Build the confidence in the process, not just in the result."

It was simple advice, but it made sense. That weekend, we ditched the baseball and brought out a tennis ball instead. I took the pressure off, told my son we were just going to have fun and focus on catching something smaller. No stakes, no expectations. We spent an afternoon tossing it back and forth, laughing, and, slowly, his confidence returned. The following week at practice, he caught his first fly ball.

Asking for help as a parent doesn't come naturally to me, but that experience reminded me that we're all in this together. We don't have to have all the answers, and sometimes, leaning on others is what makes us stronger. Just like I've been there for other parents, there's no shame in reaching out when you're the one in need of support.

Chapter 14: Stitch It All Together

As we come to the end of this journey, the challenge isn't just in understanding each chapter's lessons, but in weaving them together into a cohesive approach to parenting. Parenting isn't a collection of isolated strategies, but a dynamic and evolving process. Each principle, each story, and each piece of advice I've shared throughout this book builds on the others. Let's take a moment to stitch it all together and reflect on how everything connects, from becoming a parent, to guiding your child through life's challenges, to the ultimate goal: raising strong, net they rely on during the more challenging times.

Chapter 5 then builds on the concept of presence by adding an element of play. Playfulness and silliness aren't just about fun—they're about creating a safe environment where creativity thrives and bonds are strengthened. These moments of joy balance the harder lessons, like setting boundaries or enforcing consequences, by showing your child that discipline and fun can coexist. Children are far more willing to listen and learn when they know their parent values their joy as much as their growth.

Discipline and Empowerment: Saying "No" and "Yes"

Chapters 6 and 7 represent the dual forces of parenting: discipline and empowerment. Chapter 6 focused on the importance of setting boundaries and teaching children to navigate limits. The "no" moments are often the hardest but most essential. They teach responsibility, patience, and resilience—qualities that echo throughout their lives, from how they handle conflict to how they respond to adversity. When we give children the structure they need, we are preparing them for a world full of rules, expectations, and challenges.

But, as we discussed in Chapter 7, balance is key. It's just as important to say "yes" and empower children to explore, take risks, and learn through trial and error. Letting them get messy, make mistakes, or even get a little hurt helps them build confidence and independence. Just as we instill boundaries, we also need to give them room to grow, to test their limits in safe ways. This ties directly to the lessons in Chapter 10, where we talk about the big struggle of balancing freedom and safety. Both the "yes" and the "no" moments are necessary in preparing a child for the real world, where they will face both opportunity and restriction, and need the confidence and wisdom to navigate both.

The Power of Choice and Social Skills

In Chapter 9, we introduced the Choice Method—a tool that can transform everyday power struggles into opportunities for growth. Offering choices gives children a sense of control while guiding them toward appropriate behavior. It's a simple, powerful strategy that reduces conflict and encourages cooperation, while still enforcing boundaries. This concept of choice ties into earlier chapters on discipline and empowerment, showing how both can coexist. It also relates to Chapter 8, where we talk about social skill building. Giving children choices helps them learn decision-making, accountability, and negotiation skills—essential abilities for navigating social dynamics.

As parents, we can guide our children through difficult moments by giving them the tools to think critically and make decisions. Whether it's choosing between broccoli or carrots, or handling conflict with siblings, the ability to make choices is what empowers children to thrive socially and emotionally.

The Bigger Picture: Community and Connection

Chapter 13 explored the importance of community in parenting. Just as we align with our partners, we need to lean on other parents, teachers, and mentors in our lives. Parenting doesn't happen in isolation, and the lessons we've covered throughout this book become even stronger when supported by a network of like-minded individuals. In Chapter 12, we discussed aligning with your partner, but community extends beyond just the two of you. The village that helps raise your child offers perspectives, support, and reinforcement of the values you're working to instill at home. It's another layer of the trust we want our children to feel—not just in us, but in the world around them.

Stitching It All Together: A Holistic Approach

So, how do we stitch it all together? Parenting is not about mastering one thing at a time, but about balancing many moving parts. From discipline to empowerment, from presence to play, each chapter represents a vital piece of the puzzle. It's about teaching children to be confident yet humble, independent yet connected, disciplined yet free-spirited. We guide them through their formative years, knowing that there

will be ups and downs, but trusting that the principles we lay out
will ultimately lead them to become well-rounded,
compassionate individuals.

In the end, parenting is about love and trust—two forces that,
when balanced, can create a foundation strong enough to
support a child through anything life throws their way. Whether
it's the simple act of offering choices, the deeper connection
formed through presence, or the strong boundaries set with
discipline, every moment is a teaching moment. Every decision
we make is a thread in the fabric of our children's lives.

The goal is not to be perfect. The goal is to be there, to be
present, to guide, and to love. To create a safe place for your
children to grow, make mistakes, and ultimately, flourish.

And that's the essence of
Parenting with Purpose
—a journey that is complex, challenging, and deeply rewarding.
The principles we've discussed are not one-size-fits-all solutions
but adaptable tools to help you navigate the ever-changing
landscape of parenthood. My hope is that, as you move forward,
you'll continue to embrace both the joys and struggles of this
incredible journey, knowing that every moment, every choice,
and every "yes" or "no" helps to shape the extraordinary
individuals your children are becoming.

In the end, parenting is about showing up with love, patience, and a willingness to learn alongside your child. It's not about being perfect, but about being present. It's about knowing when to say "yes," when to say "no," and when to simply listen. As you navigate the inevitable ups and downs, trust in the foundation you've built—one made of laughter, discipline, trust, and compassion. The greatest gift we can give our children is ourselves: our time, our presence, and our unwavering belief in their potential. The journey is never easy, but it's always worth it, and with every step, you're helping shape a future filled with possibility.

Quotes for Inspiration

1. On Presence & Time:

- "Children spell love T-I-M-E." –
Dr. Anthony P. Witham

- Emphasizes the idea that being present is the most important gift parents can give their children.

2. On Empowering Children & Building Self-Esteem:

- "There is no better gift to a child than self-esteem." –
Barbara Johnson

- Highlights the importance of nurturing a child's confidence, a key concept in empowering children.

3. On Play and Silliness:

- "Play is the highest form of research." –
Albert Einstein

- Supports the idea that play is essential to a child's development, as explored in the chapter on play and silliness.

4. On Discipline and Boundaries:

- "To bring up a child in the way he should go, travel that way yourself once in a while." –
Josh Billings

o

Encourages leading by example, a principle discussed in relation to discipline and teaching values.

5. On Building Trust and Open Communication:

o

"The best way to make children good is to make them happy." – *Oscar Wilde*

o

Trust and happiness go hand-in-hand, reinforcing the idea that fostering open communication with your child builds a strong relationship.

6. On Struggles in Parenting:

o

"There is no such thing as a perfect parent, so just be a real one." –
Sue Atkins

o

Supports the notion that parenting is a constant learning process, emphasizing the authenticity required when balancing discipline, safety, and freedom.

7. On Letting Kids Take Risks and Learn:

○

"It is not what you do for your children, but what you have taught them to do for themselves that will make them successful human beings." -
Ann Landers

○

Reinforces the idea that empowering children by allowing them to make mistakes and learn is crucial.

8. On Trust and Running to You, Not Away:

○

"The most important thing that parents can teach their children is how to get along without them." -
Frank A. Clark

○

This speaks to the goal of creating trust and resilience, so your children always feel they can come to you, no matter what.

9. On Partnership in Parenting:

○

"Behind every young child who believes in themselves is a parent who believed first." -

o

Reflects the importance of parental alignment in belief and approach, discussed in the chapters on co-parenting and building a solid foundation.

10.On the Role of a Parent as a Hero and Guide:

- "A father is someone you look up to no matter how tall you grow." –
Unknown

- Captures the essence of being a hero and protector in your child's eyes, as explored in the chapters on the father's role.

The End.